Beating the Enemy: How Vitamin D Could Help Fight Covid-19

Shirley Amy BSc.

Beating the Enemy: How Vitamin D Could Help Fight Covid-19, London, England

PR Enquiries: beatingthecoronavirusenemy@gmail.com

Copyright © 2020 Shirley Amy BSc.

ISBN: 978-1-71688-266-1

A CIP catalog record for this book is available from The British Library

DISCLAIMER

The content in this book is intended for informational purposes only. The information and ideas are not in any way meant to be prescriptive without the consent of an individual's medical physician. Nothing recorded herein is intended to diagnose, treat, cure or prevent any form of disease. The information presented is in no way whatsoever intended to be a substitute for medical advice, or as a replacement for a medically approved treatment or diet. The suggestions that are given may not be suitable for people of certain ages, with certain conditions, diagnosed or otherwise.

This book is compiled to provide a spectrum of information about vitamin D, and is designed to give readers a broad outlook. It is not intended to be complete or exhaustive. Every individual is biochemically, metabolically, physically and psychologically unique, with their own genetic traits, social worlds, and life experiences. Therefore, only a medically qualified physician should diagnose specific medical conditions which relate to each individual reader. A medically qualified physician should be consulted in person to examine the individual, look at their medical history, and make the necessary tests in relation to any health problems and concerns.

Taking certain supplements (including vitamin D), can interfere with the absorption of some drugs. It is therefore, vital to discuss this with your medical physician before taking them. Always follow the instructions of your medical physician and the manufacturer (your medical physician's instructions should supersede the instructions given by the manufacturer).

If you are under the care of a medical physician or other qualified healthcare practitioner, and receive advice contrary to information provided within this book, your medical physician's or other qualified medical practitioner's advice should be followed, as it is based on your unique characteristics.

If you are suffering from any medical complaint, disease, health problem or special condition, are pregnant, breastfeeding; or on medication, homeopathic remedies, or natural or synthetic supplements, always check with an appropriately qualified medical physician that there are no contra-indications to any form of: diet, supplementation, activity or lifestyle change, you may wish to pursue. It must be stressed that everyone is unique, and medical conditions as well as age and various other factors, must be taken into consideration.

Before you decide to start taking a vitamin D supplement, it is recommended that you first have a consultation with your medical physician. This is due to a number of potential interactions. These include, but are not limited to: "aluminum, anticonvulsants, atorvastatin, calcipotriene, Cholestyramine (Prevalite), Cytochrome P450 3A4 (CYP3A4) substrates, Digoxin (Lanoxin), Diltiazem (Cardizem, Tiazac), Orlistat (Xenical, Alli), Thiazide diuretics, steroids, stimulant laxatives, and Verapamil (Verelan, Calan)" [1].

Reference:

[1]. The Mayo Clinic (2017). "Vitamin D."

https://www.mayoclinic.org/drugs-supplements-vitamin-d/art-20363792

Further, a list of vitamin D3 (cholecalciferol) drug interactions can be found at the drugs.com website page.

https://www.drugs.com/drug-interactions/cholecalciferol,vitamin-d3.html

If you require further information on vitamin D product suitability and contra-indications, discuss this with your medical physician who has a record of your medical history, and is familiar with any diseases you are suffering from, and any medication you are taking.

If you suffer from any form of illness or disease, and you wish to take up any dietary suggestions to increase the amount of vitamin D you receive, you must have the approval of your medical physician. Consuming too much vitamin D from food or supplements can result in serious illness and disease. Moreover, various foods may not be suitable for everyone. If you develop a serious disease while taking vitamin D, it is vital to have the approval of your medical physician if you wish to continue.

Should you decide to use any of the suggestions within this book, it is at your sole discretion and risk. The author and publisher expressly disclaim responsibility for: injuries or illness or any possible consequences arising from any dietary change, action or application of supplements both natural and non-natural, spending time in the sun (both with and without sunblock), or use of any other information contained herein.

The statements relating to the quality of supplements have not been evaluated by the food and drug administration of the US or any country, and are not intended to diagnose, treat, cure or prevent any disease.

The benefits of all nutritional supplements, and all categories and types of food, vary greatly in regard to the effects they have on each individual. Moreover, everyone reacts differently. Any noted or researched benefits or disadvantages that are written about herein, are subject to change and variation, and it is important for readers to check current research via an appropriate specialist. The author and publisher make no representations either expressed or implied, with regard to the usefulness, accuracy, completeness or feasibility of information contained within this book.

Information within this book is not meant to encourage the treatment of ill health, disease or other medical problems by lay people. Never ignore professional medical advice, or delay in seeking it, due to something you have read in this book.

Any application of any information given inside this book, is at the reader's sole risk. The suggestions written about in this book are only applicable to suitable individuals who have had approval by their medical physician, and who are 18 years of age, or over.

The author and publisher do not accept liability for inaccurate information, copyright or trademark infringement, or mistakes which may have inadvertently been made. The author and publisher have endeavored to ensure that the external websites given for reference are correct and running at the time of publication, and do not accept responsibility if this is not the case, and cannot take accountability as to the website's content. The best advice is to regularly check the websites listed in this book, for updates.

dedication: This book is dedicated to everyone around the globe from infants to seniors, who have lost their lives to the invisible enemy, Covid-19.

Also, a huge thank you and salute to all the wonderful front-line workers including hospital and care home staff, ambulance crews, security personnel, and the delivery people, who put their lives on the line to help save us...

Shirley Amy

INDEX

Page

Foreword

Chapter 1 - Making Sure You Get Enough Vitamin D.....................................1

Chapter 2 - Sunny Side Up.........…...6

Chapter 3 - The Multiple Benefits of Vitamin D...............................…...12

Chapter 4 - Foods Which Boost Our Vitamin D Levels.............................16

Chapter 5 - The Benefits of Vitamin D Supplement.........…....................18

Putting it All Together..22

FOREWORD

"An estimated 1 billion people worldwide, across all ethnicities and age groups, have a <u>vitamin D deficiency</u>" [1]

Beating Covid-19 and similar enemies that will confront us in the future, is in our own hands, and we all have a positive role to play to help protect ourselves, our families, our loved ones, and the population at large.

As Marie Curie said: "Nothing in life is to be feared, it is only to be understood. Now is the time to understand more, so that we may fear less." Indeed, we all have to understand - but this is not always easy with the rapidly evolving scientific research and advice. People are confused...

On a positive front, all over the world, we have great scientific minds, altruistic researchers who never give up, and state-of-the art research institutes. We are approaching the pinnacle of new innovation, and are amassing new clinical knowledge and data for epidemiology models, all the time. Hopefully, in the not too distant future, top scientists and institutions will collaborate for the greater good.

Many people have tried to find out as much as possible about the clear and present danger of Covid-19. - They have looked at what measures they can take to ward it off aside from wearing a mask and protective glasses and gloves, keeping their hands sanitized, regularly cleaning surfaces they come into contact with, practicing social distancing, isolating, and so on. But we must also make sure that our immune system stands the best chance of winning - which is what this book is all about.

Beating the Enemy: How Vitamin D Could Help in the Fight Against Covid-19, adds another vital dimension to our armor. It is based on a foundation of science-backed research on the importance of vitamin D, and the link between vitamin D and our immunity with respect to Covid-19. It includes insights and advice from global leaders such as Harvard Health, Harvard Nutrition, Yale Medicine, and the National Institutes of Health (NIH).

Further, this book serves as a guide for you to ensure that you are getting adequate levels of vitamin D through diet and/or supplements, without having to be over exposed to UVB light. And as vitamin D has been proved to ameliorate a plethora of common conditions and diseases, this will not only help in the battle against Covid-19, it can also empower and regenerate our health.

Reference

[1]. Rathish Nair and Arun Maseeh "Vitamin D: The "sunshine" vitamin."
J Pharmacol Pharmacother. 2012 Apr-Jun; 3(2): 118–126.
https://www.ncbi.nlm.nih.gov/pmc/articles/PMC3356951/

Chapter 1

MAKING SURE YOU GET ENOUGH VITAMIN D

"Vitamin D linked to low virus death rate, study finds" [1]

Firstly - a warm sunny welcome to Chapter 1. - This is where the connection between Vitamin D and Covid-19 is explained in easy to understand language that can help you appreciate the importance of this potentially crucial vitamin for yourself and your loved ones.

As the Harvard Nutrition Source notes: "Vitamin D is both a nutrient we eat, and a hormone our bodies make" [2]. We can obtain it via sunshine, food, and a vitamin D supplement. It has a massive impact on our immune system - but the bad news is that we are not all getting enough of it. In fact: "Worldwide, an estimated 1 billion people have inadequate levels of vitamin D in their blood, and deficiencies can be found in all ethnicities and age groups" [2].

"Vitamin D shown to protect against acute respiratory infections, & older adults, the group most deficient in vitamin D, are also the ones most seriously affected by COVID-19" [1]

The good news, however, is that if we need to, we can easily boost our body's vitamin D level, so that we are getting the recommended amount. - And this is especially important now, as research in relation to the current pandemic, has shown that: "Patients with severe [vitamin D] deficiency, are twice as likely to experience major [Covid-19] complications" [1]; and: "Vitamin D strengthens our [first line of immunity], our innate immunity, which involves various nonspecific defense mechanisms going into action immediately, or within hours of an antigen entering our body], thus preventing an overactive immune response [1]. Note: an antigen refers to: any substance such as Covid-19, that drives our immune system to manufacture antibodies against it.

Cytokine Storms

"Vitamin D regulates the response of white blood cells, preventing them from releasing too many inflammatory cytokines" [6]

Covid-19, influenza, as well as other respiratory diseases brought about by coronaviruses such as SARS and MERS, can be fatal if our body's immune system malfunctions and overreacts, causing what is known as a cytokine storm. - This 'storm' occurs if an excessive number of cytokines (signalling molecules) are released in a part of our body, such as our lungs, and then generate high levels of inflammation (which may be fatal) [3]. In fact: "these storms can be more deadly than the original virus the body is fighting" [4]. A good analogy is putting your foot on the accelerator with a lot of superglue on the sole of your shoe...

Ultimately, a cytokine storm generates: "high fever, excessive leakiness of blood vessels, blood clotting inside the body, extremely low blood pressure, lack of oxygen and excess acidity of the blood, and build-up of fluids in the lungs" [5]. In fact, our body turns against us, and becomes our enemy, as white blood cells are instructed to inflame and attack our healthy tissue. This leads to Multiple Organ Dysfunction Syndrome: "failure of the lungs, heart, liver, intestines, kidneys, and genitals. This may worsen and shutdown the lungs (Acute Respiratory Distress Syndrome), due to the formation of a so-called hyaline membrane, composed of debris of proteins and dead cells, lining the lungs, which makes absorption of oxygen difficult" [5]. To that end, the largest percentage of deaths are down to respiratory failure [5].

Of note, cytokine storms may be the reason why some individuals experience a serious reaction to coronaviruses, while others only get mild symptoms. It could also explain why youngsters are far less affected - their acquired immune system, AKA adaptive immune system (which is our immune system's second line of defense), is not as developed, and thus generates decreased levels of inflammation-driving molecules (cytokines) [3].

Shining a Spotlight on Recent Research

<u>Study 1</u>

Headed by a team at one of America's leading private research institutions, Northwestern University, a statistical analysis involving research taken from hospitals and clinics across 10 countries: the US, UK, Switzerland, Spain, South Korea, Iran, Italy, Germany, France and China, was undertaken to determine any possible connection between vitamin D and Covid-19. The team's inspiration for the project came about after they saw unexplained differences in the Covid-19 death rates from country to country [6].

Putting the Pieces Together

After extensive examination, the scientists discovered: "a correlation between low vitamin D levels and hyperactive immune systems. Vitamin D strengths innate immunity and prevents overactive immune responses. This finding could explain several mysteries, including why children are unlikely to die from COVID-19" [6].

Further, the research shows that countries such as the UK, Spain and Italy, which have suffered high death rates from Covid-19: "had lower levels of vitamin D compared to patients in countries that were not as severely affected" [6]. At first glance, this may seem somewhat strange, as many regions in Spain and Italy are renowned for their hot sunny climate. - But all will be explained later...

Going back to the cytokine storm (the overreaction of the body's immune system): Dr. Vadim Backman, the study's lead researcher, states that it: "can severely damage lungs and lead to acute respiratory distress syndrome and death in patients. This is what seems to kill a majority of COVID-19 patients, not the destruction of the lungs by the virus itself. It is the complications from the misdirected fire from the immune system" [6].

"Previous observational studies have reported an association between low levels of vitamin D & susceptibility to acute respiratory tract infections" [1]

Dr Backman, believes vitamin D not only boosts our innate immune system (the first part of our body to detect invaders such as viruses, parasites, bacteria and toxins), but also prevents our immune system from becoming dangerously hyperactive. He notes: "This means that having healthy levels of vitamin D could protect patients against severe complications, including death, from COVID-19" [6].

Study 2

Another study, this time headed by Dr Lee Smith of the Anglia Ruskin University, and Mr Petre Cristian Ilie, lead urologist of Queen Elizabeth Hospital King's Lynn NHS Foundation Trust, uncovered: "an association between low average levels of vitamin D and high numbers of COVID-19 cases and mortality rates across 20 European countries" [1].

Other Recent Studies

Researchers in Indonesian analyzed 780 documented cases of COVID-19, and determined that: "most patients who died had vitamin D levels below normal" [7].

Moreover, scientists in Ireland conducted an evaluation of European population studies and vitamin D levels, and found that nations with: "high rates of vitamin D deficiency, also had higher death rates from COVID-19. Those researchers asked the government to raise the vitamin D recommendations" [8].

Regions That Have High & Low Levels of Vitamin D

As most people are all too aware, sadly, both Spain and Italy have experienced high death rates due to COVID-19. Interestingly, this particular research study indicates that both nations: "have lower average vitamin D levels than most northern European countries. This is partly because people in southern Europe, particularly the elderly, avoid strong sun, while skin pigmentation also reduces natural vitamin D synthesis" [1].

So Which Countries Have the Highest Average Levels of Vitamin D?

Northern Europe has been shown to have the highest average levels of vitamin D. Indeed: "Scandinavian nations are among the countries with the lowest number of COVID-19 cases and mortality rates per head of population in Europe" [1]. This is down to the: "consumption of cod liver oil and vitamin D supplements, and possibly less sun avoidance" [1].

Dr Lee Smith, from the Anglia Ruskin University, noted that: "A previous study found that 75% of people in institutions such as hospitals and care homes, were severely deficient in vitamin D" [1]. This could potentially explain the terrible number of Covid-19 deaths in care homes.

Comment

Although the research which I have reported on in this chapter shows clear results, it must be stated that the studies were subject to limitations. For example: 1. The number of Covid-19 cases in each nation was affected by the number of tests that were carried out. And 2: Each country put different measures in place to stop the pandemic spreading.

Moreover, correlation does not always mean causation. Therefore, further research by top institutions is needed. Fortunately, at the time of writing, at least 8 studies evaluating vitamin D's role in easing or preventing COVID-19, are listed on clinicaltrials.gov.

On the bright side, (please excuse the pun!), subject to any contra-indications you may personally have, making sure you get enough vitamin D, certainly seems to be a step in the right direction to help beat the enemy... And it is beneficial in a plethora of other ways, all of which will be listed later on in the book.

References

[1]. Science Daily (2020). "Vitamin D Linked to Low Virus Death Rate, Study Finds."

https://www.sciencedaily.com/releases/2020/05/200507131012.htm

[2]. Harvard Health. The Nutrition Source (2020). "Vitamin D."

https://www.hsph.harvard.edu/nutritionsource/vitamin-d/

[3]. George, Alison (2020). "Cytokin Storm." New Scientist.

https://www.newscientist.com/term/cytokine-storm/

[4]. Bradley, Sarah (2020). "What Is a Cytokine Storm? Doctors Explain How Some COVID-19 Patients' Immune Systems Turn Deadly." Health.

https://www.health.com/condition/infectious-diseases/coronavirus/cytokine-storm

[5]. Science Daily (2020). "How Covid-19 Kills."
https://www.sciencedaily.com/releases/2020/05/200513081810.htm

[6]. Science Daily (2020). "Vitamin D Levels Appear to Play Role in COVID-19 Mortality Rates."

https://www.sciencedaily.com/releases/2020/05/200507121353.htm

[7]. Raharusun, P. et al. (2020). "Patterns of COVID-19 Mortality and Vitamin D: An Indonesian Study." SSRN.

https://papers.ssrn.com/sol3/papers.cfm?abstract_id=3585561#references-widget

[8]. Laird. E. et al. (2020). "Vitamin D and Inflammation: Potential Implications For Severity of Covid-19." *The Irish Medical Journal*.

http://imj.ie/vitamin-d-and-inflammation-potential-implications-for-severity-of-covid-19/

Chapter 2
SUNNY SIDE UP

UV Light

The Ultraviolet (UV) light which reaches the earth's surface, comes in two different forms: UVA and UVB. These are classed according to their wavelength, and can also be distinguished by their biological activity, and the degree to which they can penetrate our skin [1].

UVB

Medium-wavelength UVB - the form we are concerned with in relation to vitamin D, is extremely biologically active, although it cannot penetrate further than the superficial layers of our skin. UVB rays are responsible for delayed tanning and burning. Moreover, UVB also intensifies skin aging, and plays a significant role in the development of skin cancer [1].

Clearly, this means that under various conditions, we must restrict the amount of time we spend outside without any sun protection. We must always be mindful that: "because ultraviolet rays can cause skin cancer, it is important to avoid excessive sun exposure, and in general, tanning beds should not be used" [2].

So How Exactly is Vitamin D Formed?

Harvard Health notes that: sunscreen stops people getting burned due to blocking out all the UVB rays they encounter. In fact: "an Australian study that's often cited, showed no difference in vitamin D between adults randomly assigned to use sunscreen one summer, and those assigned a placebo cream" [4]. Moreover, research shows that: "use of sunscreen; correctly applied sunscreen can reduce vitamin D absorption by more than 90%" [2].

"Sun-induced vitamin D synthesis is greatly influenced by season, time of day, latitude, altitude, air pollution, skin pigmentation, sunscreen use, passing through glass and plastic, & aging" [3]

So, let's take a look at the some of the factors which reduce our exposure to UVB light, and hence, the amount of vitamin D we can absorb. These comprise:

How we use sunscreen: when we apply an appropriate product correctly, it:

"can reduce vitamin D absorption by more than 90%" [2].

How we dress: wearing full clothing which covers our legs and arms, means we get less UVB exposure [4].

Going outside: only spending a limited amount of time in the open air means that we get less UVB rays [2]. Note: we cannot receive adequate UVB exposure sitting in a car, or being close to indoor windows. This is due to the fact that most car and commercial glass is manufactured to block out UVB rays [5].

The shade of our skin: people with darker skin tones derived from having higher amounts of the skin pigment, melanin, are protected to a certain degree. This is because their level of pigmentation acts as a form of natural sunscreen [2].

Advanced age: can cause changes in the skin, and decrease the levels of the steroid necessary for the formation of vitamin D3. Moreover, seniors are naturally inclined to spend more of their time indoors [2].

Where we live: during the winter months, the further away from the equator we live, the less vitamin D-producing UVB light we receive [4].

Certain medical conditions: including inflammatory bowel disease (Crohn's disease, ulcerative colitis), and other conditions which inhibit our body's normal fat digestion process. Note: as vitamin D is fat-soluble, it is dependent on our gut's ability to assimilate dietary fat [2].

Individuals who are obese: often have lower levels of vitamin D in their blood. This is because although vitamin D accrues in excess fat tissues, it is not readily available when needed for various body functions. "Conversely, blood levels of vitamin D rise when obese people lose weight" [2].

Patients who have had gastric bypass surgery: which normally involves removing the upper region of the small intestine, where vitamin D is absorbed [2].

Various medications: which impede our body's ability to absorb or convert vitamin D [6].

Certain seasons and short days: can reduce the amount of UVB rays on our skin [2].

Living above: the equator in a northern latitude, can make UVB light weaker [2].

Air quality: carbon particles derived from burning wood, fossil fuels and other matter, float in the air and absorb UVB rays, thereby decreasing the production of vitamin D. Conversely, UVB radiation is absorbed by ozone. - To that end, holes in the ozone layer which have developed due to pollution, may actually intensify vitamin D levels [4].

Living in big cities: where sunlight is blocked out by large buildings [7].

The Power of the Seasons

Here are some examples to show you just how much the seasons can affect our vitamin D uptake:

People living in regions in the northern hemisphere, for example: Bergen (Norway), Edmonton (Canada), and Boston (US), are not able to generate an adequate amount of vitamin D from sun exposure alone, for 6, 5, and 4 months of the year, respectively. Moreover, those who live in areas across the southern hemisphere, for instance: Cape Town (South Africa), and Buenos Aires (Argentina), receive far less sun-generated vitamin D during their winter months (between June and August), compared to what they can receive during their spring and summer months [2].

Can Our Body Store Vitamin D?

The answer to this is yes: our bodies can store vitamin D from our skin's exposure during our country's summertime. However, the problem is that the vitamin D store has to last for many months. So unfortunately, by the time late winter arrives, a high percentage of the population in these higher-latitude locales, are deficient in vitamin D [2].

The Use of Sunscreen

"If you are using sunshine for a vitamin D boost, you only need about 10-15 minutes in direct sun to reap the benefits. Remember, too much sun is a risk factor for skin cancer. Wear sunscreen & you'll still get your daily dose" [8]

Harvard Health notes that: sunscreen stops people getting burned due to blocking out all the UVB rays they encounter. In fact: "an Australian study that's often cited, showed no difference in vitamin D between adults randomly assigned to use sunscreen one summer, and those assigned a placebo cream" [4]. Moreover, research shows that: "use of sunscreen; correctly applied sunscreen can reduce vitamin D absorption by more than 90%" [2].

Different Levels of Sunscreen Protection

The American Cancer Society notes that: "SPF 15 sunscreens filter out about 93% of UVB rays, while SPF 30 sunscreens filter out about 97%, SPF 50 sunscreens about 98%, and SPF 100 about 99%" [9]. This means that by applying any of these, we will still receive a small amount of UVB rays, and hence some vitamin D.

Our Skin Colour

Melanin is the natural pigment in our skin which gives it its colour. It competes for UVB with the substance in our skin which stimulates our body to generate vitamin D. To that end, individuals with dark skin, generally need more UVB exposure in order to generate the same amount of vitamin D than those with light-skin [4].

Our Weight

Once vitamin D has been absorbed via our skin, or acquired from food or supplements, it is stored in our body's fat cells (because it is a fat-soluble vitamin) [3]. It then remains there in an inactive from until it is needed for specific body functions. Using a process referred to as hydroxylation, our liver and kidneys then convert this stored vitamin D into its active form (calcitriol) [11]. However, "being obese is correlated with low vitamin D levels, and being overweight may affect the bioavailability of vitamin D" [4].

Different Age Groups

Unlike the younger population: older people's skin contains lower levels of the substance which UVB light converts into the forerunner for vitamin D. "There's also experimental evidence that older people are less efficient vitamin D producers than younger people" [4].

So, What About the Risks of Solely Getting Vitamin D from Sun Exposure?

Sunshine uplifts us all, and very importantly, can endow us with vitamin D. - But there is also a dark side that can come about from too much sun exposure. Yale Medicine dermatologist, Amanda Zubek, MD, PhD., states that: "The risks that sun exposure poses just don't outweigh the benefits" [10]. Moreover, David J. Leffell, MD, Yale Medicine dermatologist and chief of Dermatologic Surgery, notes that: "The majority of people can get their vitamin D from nutritional supplements and from vitamin D-fortified foods" [11]. - You can read how to do this over the next two chapters.

So, What's the Best Advice on Protecting Ourselves Against Skin Cancer?

"Since skin cancer is the most common form of cancer in the US, it's important to practice sun safety before heading outdoors " [10]

Yale Medicine endocrinologist, and director of the Yale Medicine's Bone Center, Karl Insogna, MD, writes very succinctly, and offers excellent advice. He notes: "Just being outdoors, you get a fair amount of sun exposure and some sun-related generation of vitamin D. Because skin cancer, particularly melanoma, can be such a devastating disease, it's best to use sunblock when outdoors in strong sunlight for any prolonged length of time. Because this may limit the amount of vitamin D you get from sun exposure, make sure your diet includes sources of vitamin D from foods or supplements" [11].

For more information on sun protection, visit the websites of The American Cancer Society and Yale Medicine. They are shown in the following reference list, and are numbered [9] and [10], respectively.

References

[1]. The World Health Organization (2020). "UV Radiation."

https://www.who.int/uv/faq/whatisuv/en/index2.html

[2]. Harvard Health. The Nutrition Source (2020). "Vitamin D."

https://www.hsph.harvard.edu/nutritionsource/vitamin-d/

[3]. Wacker M, Holick MF. Sunlight and Vitamin D: A Global Perspective for Health. *Dermatoendocrinol*. 2013;5(1):51-108.

https://www.ncbi.nlm.nih.gov/pmc/articles/PMC3897598/

[4]. Harvard Health Publishing (N.d.). "6 Things You Should Know About Vitamin D."

https://www.health.harvard.edu/staying-healthy/6-things-you-should-know-about-vitamin-d

[5]. Rabin, C.R. (2019). "Does Sunlight Through Glass Provide Vitamin E?" *The Times*.

https://www.nytimes.com/2019/02/08/well/live/does-sunlight-through-glass-provide-vitamin-d.html

[6]. Medline Plus (2019). "Vitamin D Deficiency."

https://medlineplus.gov/vitaminddeficiency.html

[7]. Healthline (2017). "The Benefits of Vitamin D."

https://www.healthline.com/health/food-nutrition/benefits-vitamin-d

[8]. Livewell Unitypoint Health (2020). "How to Spot a Vitamin D Deficiency."

https://www.unitypoint.org/livewell/article.aspx?id=ca7f4766-8ba8-43a2-bbe7-0ef9efab5c6d

[9]. American Cancer Society (2019). "How Do I Protect Myself from Ultraviolet (UV) Rays?"

https://www.cancer.org/healthy/be-safe-in-sun/uv-protection.html

[10]. Moriarty, C. (2017). "9 Ways to Lower Skin Cancer Risk." Yale Medicine.

https://www.yalemedicine.org/stories/9-ways-to-lower-skin-cancer-risk/

[11]. Moriarty, C. (2018). "Vitamin D Myths 'D'-bunked." Yale Medicine.

https://www.yalemedicine.org/stories/vitamin-d-myths-debunked/

Chapter 3

THE MULTIPLE BENEFITS OF VITAMIN D

"Vitamin D helps support a healthy brain, heart, teeth & lungs. It keeps our immune system strong & can help regulate insulin levels. It also keeps our energy levels up and enhances our mood" [1]

Aside from our battle against Covid-19, Vitamin D is also crucial for our bones' mineralization and regeneration, not to mention many functions which do not involve our skeleton, especially those involving our cardiovascular, endocrine and immune systems [2]. To that end, if you find you are deficient in vitamin D, and rectify the situation to bring it up to an optimum level, then you will score a double whammy for your health and wellness.

In a nutshell, vitamin D is involved in:

Promoting healthy teeth and bones [3]. "Vitamin D regulates the circulating levels of calcium and phosphorus, which are the most important minerals for bone growth and maintenance. It promotes the absorption of these minerals Taking vitamin D supplements over the long-term may lessen the risk of multiple sclerosis [5].

Adults with a serious a vitamin D deficiency due to: muscle weakness, bone pain, soft bones, and loss of bone mineral content, are treated with vitamin D supplements [5].

Individuals who ingest sufficient vitamin D and calcium in their diets, can slow the loss of bone minerals, reduce bone fractures, and help prevent osteoporosis [5].

Supplementing with vitamin D can treat and prevent rickets. (Individuals with rickets may have stunted growth, soft and weak bones, and in grave cases, skeletal deformities) [5].

Vitamin D could help lower the chances of developing the flu [4]

Vitamin D could have a vital role in staving off depression and regulating mood. "In one study, scientists found that people with depression who received vitamin D supplements noticed an improvement" [4].

When studying individuals with fibromyalgia, researchers found that: "vitamin D deficiency was more common in those experiencing anxiety and depression" [4]. On the subject of weight loss, research shows that: "people taking a daily calcium and vitamin D supplement, were able to lose more weight than subjects taking a placebo. The scientists said the extra calcium and vitamin D had an appetite-suppressing effect" [4].

Vitamin D Deficiency

The Harvard Nutrition Source notes that: "a vitamin D deficiency [also known as hypovitaminosis D, or low Vitamin D], may occur from a lack in the diet, poor absorption; or having a metabolic need for higher amounts. If one is not eating enough vitamin D, and does not receive enough ultraviolet sun exposure over an extended period, a deficiency may arise" [6].

Unfortunately, many people with a vitamin D deficiency do not realize that they actually have one. - This is due to the fact that the symptoms are usually very subtle, and they could easily be caused by something else [1]. So, let's take a look at some of them. These include:

Fatigue or tiredness

Pain in the bones

Joint pain

Muscle pain

Being in an unpleasant mood

Low energy levels

Being ill more frequently

Feeling anxious

Getting irritable

Gaining weight Loosing hair [1].

How Can I Test for Vitamin D Deficiency?

A simple blood test which will give you the results you need, can either be booked online with a reputable company, or via your doctor. Unity Point LiveWell states that: "The most accurate way to measure how much vitamin D is in your body, is the 25-hydroxy vitamin D blood test. Many experts place the ideal level between 40 and 80 ng/mL with levels below 20 ng/mL as deficient." [1]. Note ng stands for nanograms. Be sure to check with your insurance company to see if they will cover a vitamin D test with your doctor. If not, an online test will be far cheaper [1].

Understanding the Measurements

Levels [for 25-hydroxy vitamin D] are described in either: nanomoles per liter (nmol/L), or nanograms per milliliter (ng/mL), where 1 nmol/L = 0.4 ng/mL" [7].

What Level Should I Have?

The NIH (National Institutes of Health) notes that: "In general, levels below 30 nmol/L (12 ng/mL) are too low for bone or overall health, and levels above 125 nmol/L (50 ng/mL) are probably too high. Levels of 50 nmol/L or above (20 ng/mL or above) are sufficient for most people" [7].

References

[1]. Unity Point Health LiveWell (2019). "How to Spot a Vitamin D Deficiency."

https://www.unitypoint.org/livewell/article.aspx?id=ca7f4766-8ba8-43a2-bbe7-0ef9efab5c6d

[2]. Oregon State University, The Linus Pauling Institute (2017). "Vitamin D."

https://lpi.oregonstate.edu/mic/vitamins/vitamin-D

[3]. Ware, M. (2019). "What Are the Health Benefits of Vitamin D?." Medical News Today.

https://www.medicalnewstoday.com/articles/161618#deficiency [4].

Healthline (2017). "The Benefits of Vitamin D."

https://www.healthline.com/health/food-nutrition/benefits-vitamin-d

[5]. The Mayo Clinic (2017). "Vitamin D."

https://www.mayoclinic.org/drugs-supplements-vitamin-d/art-20363792

[6]. Harvard School of Public Health. The Nutrition Source (2020). "Vitamin D."

https://www.hsph.harvard.edu/nutritionsource/vitamin-d/

[7]. National Institutes of Health (NIH) (2020). "Vitamin D Fact Sheet for Consumers."

https://ods.od.nih.gov/factsheets/VitaminD-Consume

Chapter 4

FOODS WHICH BOOST OUR VITAMIN D LEVELS

Vitamin D3 has a unique metabolism, as it is mainly generated via synthesis in the skin, brought about by sunlight (UVB radiation). Conversely, receiving vitamin D from nutrition, plays a comparatively minor role [1]. However, as you have already read, we cannot always rely on getting sufficient vitamin D from the sun. Further, due to the clear and present danger of being susceptible to skin cancer, we do need to wear sun cream with a decent sun protection factor, according to our needs.

Vitamin D is classed into two main categories: vitamin D2 (ergocalciferol), which is derived from plants and fungi; and vitamin D3 (cholecalciferol), which is found in animal food. Both categories raise the level of vitamin D in our blood, and as they occur naturally in certain foods, we can easily add some to our daily menus to boost our vitamin D levels, and avoid a deficiency [2].

The Low Down

David J. Leffell, MD, a Yale Medicine dermatologist, & chief of Dermatologic Surgery, notes: "The majority of people can get their vitamin D from nutritional supplements & from vitamin D-fortified foods" [2].

Only a handful of foods are naturally abundant in vitamin D3. The Harvard Nutrition Source states that: "the best sources are the flesh of fatty fish (salmon, tuna, mackerel, swordfish, etc.), and fish liver oils (e.g., cod liver oil). Smaller amounts are found in free range egg yolks, cheese, and beef liver, [and] certain mushrooms (including those exposed to UV light), contain some vitamin D2" [3].

However, as we do not usually eat these foods in sufficient quantities, more and more manufacturers of various products such as: orange juice, cereal, bread, dairy milk, margarine, and vegan milk, yogurt and cheese, fortify their products with vitamin D2 and D3. In fact, this practice started out way back in the 1930s, when some manufacturers voluntarily enriched their foods with vitamin D to help lower the frequency of nutritional rickets [2]. Indeed, systematic vitamin D food fortification both then and now, has been shown to be successful [1].

The NIH (National Institutes of Health) states that our nutritional requirements: "should be met primarily from foods... Foods in nutrient-dense forms contain essential vitamins and minerals and also dietary fiber and other naturally occurring substances that may have positive health effects" [4]. Moreover, dietary supplements, and foods which have been fortified with vitamin D, could be beneficial [4].

Higher Risks of Deficiency

"People who cannot tolerate or do not eat milk, eggs, & fish, such as those with a lactose intolerance or who follow a vegan diet, are at higher risk of a deficiency" [3]

When it comes to nutrient deficiencies, the NIH note that these are normally: "the result of dietary inadequacy, impaired absorption and use, increased requirement, or increased excretion. A vitamin D deficiency can occur when usual intake is lower than recommended levels over time, exposure to sunlight is limited, the kidneys cannot convert 25(OH)D to its active form, or absorption of vitamin D from the digestive tract is inadequate" [4]. Diets which are deficient in Vitamin D, are linked with veganism, ovo-vegetarianism (no dairy consumption); being lactose intolerant, or having a milk allergy [4].

If you do have a vitamin D deficiency, then your doctor will be able to recommend a suitable vitamin D supplement (subject to any contra- indications). Further, a registered nutritionist should be able to give you a personalized diet plan, which could help bump up your vitamin D intake.

Vegans

Of note, if you are vegan, supplements are readily available in D2 form (which is derived from fungi and algae), so you do not have to take the D3 (animal derived) form.

References

[1]. Pilz S, März W. et al. "Rationale and Plan for Vitamin D Food Fortification: A Review and Guidance Paper." Front Endocrinol (Lausanne). (2018); 9:373.

https://www.ncbi.nlm.nih.gov/pmc/articles/PMC6056629/

[2]. Moriarty, Colleen (2018). "Vitamin D Myths 'D'-bunked." Yale Medicine. https://www.yalemedicine.org/stories/vitamin-d-myths-debunked

[3]. Harvard Source of Public Health. The Nutrition Source (2020). "Vitamin D." https://www.hsph.harvard.edu/nutritionsource/vitamin-d/

[4]. National Institutes of Health (NIH) (2020). "Vitamin D Fact Sheet For Consumers." https://ods.od.nih.gov/factsheets/VitaminD-Consumer/

Chapter 5

THE BENEFITS OF VITAMIN D SUPPLEMENTS

Along with sunshine and certain foods, a third route to boosting our vitamin D level, is taking supplements in pill, capsule, or liquid/spray form. Vitamin D supplements come in two types: vitamin D2 (ergocalciferol or pre-vitamin D) and vitamin D3 (cholecalciferol). Vitamin D2 is derived from plants, and can be found in fortified food and some supplements. Conversely, Vitamin D3 is naturally produced by our bodies, and is present in animal food [1].

According to Yale Medicine, supplements: "are generally recommended for people with fat absorption issues, lactose intolerance, milk allergies, as well as for people with darker skin tones or with certain medical conditions that prevent them from going outdoors" [2].

How Much Vitamin D Should I Take?

The NIH (National Institutes of Health), note that the amount of vitamin D we need every day, is dependent on our age. The recommended average daily amounts listed in micrograms (mcg) and International Units (IU), are as follows:

Teenagers age 14 to 18 years old: 15 mcg (600 IU)

Adults age 19 to 70 years old: 15 mcg (600 IU)

Adults age 71 and over: 20 mcg (800 IU)

Pregnant & Breastfeeding Women: 15 mcg (600 IU)

(Reference: NIH [3]).

Liquid or Capsules?

Although both forms of vitamin D supplements generate the same health benefits, the advantage of liquid vitamins, is that due to their superior bio-availability, our bodies do not have to brake them down and digest them. Moreover, this form of vitamin D is the best choice for anyone with low stomach acid and impaired digestion [4].

Better Absorbed With a Meal

As vitamin D is fat-soluble, it does not dissolve in water. Therefore, it is best absorbed in our bloodstream at the time we consume high-fat foods. To that end, taking vitamin D supplements with food is the best practice [4]. Nutritious sources of fat which can help vitamin D absorption, include: eggs, full-fat dairy products, seeds, nuts, and avocados [5].

What the Research Says

One research study indicates that: "17 people taking vitamin D with the largest meal of the day, increased vitamin D blood levels by about 50% after just 2–3 months. [Further], another study involving 50 older adults consuming vitamin D alongside a fat-heavy meal, increased vitamin D blood levels by 32% after 12 hours compared to a fat-free meal" [5].

So, What is the Best Time of Day?

Some people may like to take their vitamin D in the morning with breakfast, while others may prefer lunchtime. However, as: "anecdotal reports assert that supplementing with vitamin D at nighttime may interfere with sleep" [5], it may be better to just stick with taking it with breakfast or lunch.

Being Smart About E

The Michael and Lee Bell Professor of Women's Health at Harvard Medical School, Dr Joann E. Manson, has published some much needed, easy to follow guidelines, which are designed to help people take vitamin D supplements safely. These include: Watching Your Numbers. She notes: "If you're taking a vitamin D supplement, you probably don't need more than 600 to 800 IU per day, which is adequate for most people. Some people may need a higher dose, including those with a bone health disorder and those with a condition that interferes with the absorption of vitamin D or calcium. Unless your doctor recommends it, avoid taking more than 4,000 IU per day, which is considered the safe upper limit" [6]. Note: if you are taking a multivitamin or other supplement which includes vitamin D, be sure to add the IUs to your total intake.

Shopping for Supplements

As Yale Medicine suggests, always shop for vitamin D supplements that: "offer the daily recommended allowance (RDA) you need for your age bracket: for most healthy people, it's 600 IU per day, but for people over age 70 who need a little more - it's about 800 IU. That's because, as people age (women after menopause, in particular), they less efficiently synthesize vitamin D and absorb calcium" [7].

Be Sure to Tell Your Doctor

Dr Manson remarks that a substantial percentage of people are taking high-dose supplements on their own volition, and may not have informed their physicians. To that end, he recommends that everyone discusses supplement use with their doctor, in order to make sure that the levels they are taking correspond to their needs. He states: "If you have a well-balanced diet, which regularly includes good sources of vitamin D, you may not need a supplement at all" [6].

Which is Better - Vitamin D2 or Vitamin D3?

When it comes to increasing our blood levels of vitamin D, it has not been fully determined whether vitamin D3 is preferable to vitamin D2. A statistical analysis which examined the results of multiple scientific studies which: "compared the effects of vitamin D2 and D3 supplements on blood levels, found that D3 supplements tended to raise blood concentrations of the vitamin more and sustained those levels longer than D2" [1]. Moreover, as vitamin D3 is naturally produced by our bodies, and found in the majority of foods which naturally incorporate vitamin D, understandably, some experts believe that this is the best source [1].

A Caution

As previously mentioned, if you are suffering from a disease, or are on pharmaceuticals, you should ensure that there are no contra-indications to taking a vitamin D supplement, by speaking with your doctor who has your medical history, and knows about any disease or illness you have, and your current medication.

A list of Vitamin D3 (cholecalciferol) Drug Interactions can be found at the following drugs.com website page. However, it is strongly advised that you still speak with your doctor prior to taking vitamin D.

https://www.drugs.com/drug-interactions/cholecalciferol,vitamin-d3.html

Moreover, even if you do not have a disease, and are not on pharmaceuticals, speak to your doctor about taking a vitamin D supplement.

Toxicity

"Vitamin D toxicity is usually caused by large doses of vitamin D supplements — not by diet or sun exposure. That's because your body regulates the amount of vitamin D produced by sun exposure, and even fortified foods don't contain large amounts of vitamin D" [8].

Symptoms include: irregular heartbeat, weight loss, anorexia; and the hardening of tissues and blood vessels derived from raised levels of calcium in the blood, which can potentially generate damage to the kidneys and heart [1].

References

[1]. Harvard School of Public Health. The Nutrition Source (2020). "Vitamin D."

https://www.hsph.harvard.edu/nutritionsource/vitamin-d/

[2]. Moriarty, Colleen (2018). "Vitamin D Myths 'D'-Bunked." Yale Medicine.

https://www.yalemedicine.org/stories/vitamin-d-myths-debunked

[3]. National Institutes of Health (NIH) (2020). "Vitamin D Fact Sheet For Consumers."

https://ods.od.nih.gov/factsheets/VitaminD-Consumer/

[4]. Ashton, J.J. (2017). "What Are the Benefits of Liquid Vitamin D-3?." SF Gate.

https://healthyeating.sfgate.com/benefits-liquid-vitamin-d3-12051.html

[5]. Link, Rachael (2018). "When Is the Best Time to Take Vitamin D? Morning or Night?" Healthline.

https://www.healthline.com/nutrition/best-time-to-take-vitamin-d#with-food

[6]. Harvard Health Publishing. Harvard Medical School (2019). "Taking Too Much Vitamin D Can Cloud Its Benefits and Create Health Risks."

https://www.health.harvard.edu/staying-healthy/taking-too-much-vitamin-d-can-cloud-its-benefits-and-create-health-risks

[7]. Moriarty, C. (2018). "Vitamin D Myths 'D'-bunked." Yale Medicine.

https://www.yalemedicine.org/stories/vitamin-d-myths-debunked/

[8]. Zeratsky, K. (2020). "What is Vitamin D Toxicity? Should I Be worried About Taking Supplements?" Mayo Clinic.

https://www.mayoclinic.org/healthy-lifestyle/nutrition-and-healthy-eating/expert-answers/vitamin-d-toxicity/faq-20058108

PUTTING IT ALL TOGETHER

As you now know, there are three ways that our bodies can get vitamin D: via the sun, from certain foods, and by taking vitamin D supplements. And as you also know, due to various reasons, many of us have a vitamin D deficiency.

You have also seen the research which shows how an optimum level of available vitamin D in our bodies could play a vital role in helping us beat the current Covid-19 enemy, and possibly similar pandemics that may come to haunt us in the future. Moreover, you are now aware that vitamin D is essential for numerous important body functions, and hence, optimum health.

With regard to calculating the sum total of the different ways we obtain vitamin D every day, i.e., via the sun and food, there are some online calculators, although this method is quite complex, as is working out how much UVB light you receive where you live. However, by making yourself familiar with the list of foods which naturally contain vitamin D, and are enriched with vitamin D, you could always add some to your meals.

Further, if after reading this book, you think that you may have a vitamin D deficiency, then you could always get a home, or doctor's surgery test. If you do need to take a vitamin D supplement, always discuss it with your doctor, who should be able to recommend one, as long as you do not have any contraindications due to a disease, illness, or any medication you are taking.

Throughout the course of this book, I have used information from some of the world's leading authorities - all of which are doing a wonderful job, which includes sending out free information about how we can attain optimum health and wellness, and thus, life our best lives. All the references I have used are at the end of every chapter; and you can explore the associated websites for further information and updates.

#QuitforCovid

"Centers for Disease Control Says COVID-19 Symptoms Worse for Smokers, E-Cigarette Users" [1]

Moreover, the American Lung Association has called for smokers to quit so they can: "immediately improve their overall health, and help prevent the most serious symptoms of COVID-19" [1]. To that end, if you do smoke, now is the time to join the countless people who have quit as a result of this invisible enemy, and potential future enemies.

Recent research findings which were published by the *New England Journal of Medicine*, indicate that: "smokers were 2.4 times more likely to have severe symptoms from COVID-19 compared to those who did not smoke" [1]. Further, the American Lung Association has stated that: "Tobacco smoke and vape emissions effects our ability to fight viruses and disrupts the immune system causing inflammation in our airways. The presence of this inflammation in the face of an additional insult like an acute disease makes it harder for our lungs to combat the invading virus and sets up the risk for severe complications of the infection" [1].

The time is now, so if you would like a helping hand, please read my book, "The Winning Way to Quit Smoking," which is free for Amazon Prime members, and is also available for purchase in Kindle and printed format from all Amazon based countries, as well as other leading distributors. It offers smokers who have not been successful at quitting, and new would-be quitters, a revolutionary, new easy holistic approach to turning their lives around, and quitting for good [2].

https://www.amazon.com/Winning-Way-Quit-Smoking-

Once you read about how your brain is controlling your addiction; like many people who have been inspired by my book, you may be able to quit right away. Alternatively, if you prefer to cut down gradually: all you have to do is to follow the protocol, and reduce your cigarette intake by just 10% a month, while systematically building up your mental and physical strength with cutting-edge holistic suggestions and supports. These include using specific de-stressing aromatherapy oils, and drinking Quit Tea [3], which relaxes you, ameliorates lung function, and helps you fight the urge to light up.

Now, getting back to this book, I wholeheartedly thank you for your interest, and I very much hope that my small contribution to fighting the herculean Covid-19 enemy, will do a lot of good, and put us all in a stronger position to protect ourselves against its current deadly force, and any future similar recurrences that could once again threaten every part of our beautiful planet and way of life.

#wewillsurvive

References

[1]. CBS Minnesota (2020). "Coronavirus Updates: CDC Says COVID-19 Symptoms Worse for Smokers, E-Cigarette Users."

https://minnesota.cbslocal.com/2020/03/31/coronavirus-updates-cdc-says-covid-19-symptoms-worse-for-smokers-e-cigarette-users/

[2]. Amy, Shirley (2012). The Winning Way to Quit Smoking.

https://www.amazon.com/Winning-Way-Quit-Smoking-ebook/dp/B007QYD98S/ref=sr_1_1?dchild=1&keywords=shirley+amy+winning+way&qid=1590515182&sr=8-1#customerReviews

[3]. The Quit Co (2020). Quit Tea & other smoking cessation products.

https://www.amazon.com/quittea

What is this life, if full of care,

We have no time to stand and stare.

No time to stand beneath the boughs
And stare as long as sheep or cows.

No time to see, when woods we pass,
Where squirrels hide their nuts in grass.

No time to see, in broad daylight,
Streams full of stars, like skies at night.

No time to turn at Beauty's glance,
And watch her feet, how they can dance.

No time to wait till her mouth can
Enrich that smile her eyes began.

A poor life this if, full of care,
We have no time to stand and stare.

Leisure, W.H. Davies, 1911